TAKE MASTERY OF YOUR HEALTH:
Understanding and Controlling Hypertension.

Dr. Robert E. Wright

Table of Contents

Chapter 1: HYPERTENSION, AN OVERVIEW

Key facts

Hypertension – or elevated blood pressure – is a serious medical condition that significantly increases the risks of heart, brain, kidney and other diseases.

•An estimated 1.28 billion adults aged 30-79 years worldwide have hypertension, most (two-thirds) living in low- and middle-income countries

•An estimated 46% of adults with hypertension are unaware that they have the condition.

•Less than half of adults (42%) with hypertension are diagnosed and treated.

•Approximately 1 in 5 adults (21%) with hypertension have it under control.

•Hypertension is a major cause of premature death worldwide.

•One of the global targets for noncommunicable diseases is to reduce the prevalence of hypertension by 33% between 2010 and 2030.

Facts About Hypertension in the United States

In 2017, the American College of Cardiology and the American Heart Association published new guidelines for hypertension management and defined high hypertension as a blood pressure at or above 130/80 mmHg. Stage 2 hypertension is defined as a blood pressure at or above 140/90 mmHg.

Blood Pressure Category	Systolic Blood Pressure	Diastolic Blood Pressure
Normal	<120 mmHg	<80 mmHg

Elevated   120-129 mmHg
                                  <80 mmHg

Hypertension

Stage 1   130-139 mmHg
                                  80-89 mmHg

Stage 2   ≥140 mmHg
                                  ≥90 mmHg

Having hypertension puts you at risk for heart disease and stroke, which are leading causes of death in the United States.

In 2020, more than 670,000 deaths in the United States had hypertension as a primary or contributing cause.

Nearly half of adults in the United States (47%, or 116 million) have hypertension, defined as a systolic blood pressure greater than 130 mmHg or a diastolic blood pressure greater than 80 mmHg or are taking medication for hypertension.

Only about 1 in 4 adults (24%) with hypertension have their condition under control.

About half of adults (45%) with uncontrolled hypertension have a blood pressure of 140/90 mmHg or higher. This includes 37 million U.S. adults.

About 34 million adults who are recommended to take medication may need it to be prescribed and to start taking it. Almost two out of three of this group (19 million) have a blood pressure of 140/90 mmHg or higher.

High blood pressure costs the United States about $131 billion each year, averaged over 12 years from 2003 to 2014.

Rates of High Blood Pressure Control Vary by Sex and Race

Uncontrolled high blood pressure is common; however, certain groups of people are more likely to have control over their high blood pressure than others.

A greater percentage of men (50%) have high blood pressure than women (44%).

High blood pressure is more common in non-Hispanic black adults (56%) than in non-Hispanic white adults (48%), non-Hispanic Asian adults (46%), or Hispanic adults (39%).

Among those recommended to take blood pressure medication, blood pressure control is higher among non-Hispanic white adults (32%) than in non-Hispanic black adults (25%), non-Hispanic Asian adults (19%), or Hispanic adults (25%).

What is hypertension?

Blood pressure is the force exerted by circulating blood against the walls of the body's arteries, the major blood vessels in the body. Hypertension is when blood pressure is too high.

Blood pressure is written as two numbers. The first **(systolic)** number represents the pressure in blood vessels when the heart contracts or beats. The second **(diastolic)** number represents the pressure in the vessels when the heart rests between beats.

Hypertension is diagnosed if, when it is measured on two different days, the systolic blood pressure readings on both days is ≥140 mmHg and/or the diastolic blood pressure readings on both days is ≥90 mmHg.

What are common symptoms of hypertension?

Hypertension is called a **"silent killer"**. Most people with hypertension are unaware of the problem because it may have no warning signs or symptoms. For this reason, it is essential that blood pressure is measured regularly.

When symptoms do occur, they can include early morning headaches, nosebleeds, irregular heart rhythms, vision changes, and buzzing in the ears. Severe hypertension can cause fatigue, nausea, vomiting, confusion, anxiety, chest pain, and muscle tremors.

The only way to detect hypertension is to have a health professional measure blood pressure. Having blood pressure measured is quick and painless. Although individuals can measure their own blood pressure using automated devices, an evaluation by a health professional is important for assessment of risk and associated conditions.

Why is hypertension an important issue in low- and middle-income countries?

The prevalence of hypertension varies across regions and country income groups. The WHO African Region has the highest prevalence of hypertension (27%) while the WHO Region of the Americas has the lowest prevalence of hypertension (18%).

The number of adults with hypertension increased from 594 million in 1975 to 1.13 billion in 2015, with the increase seen largely in low- and middle-income countries. This increase is due mainly to a rise in hypertension risk factors in those populations.

What is the WHO response?

The World Health Organization (WHO) is supporting countries to reduce hypertension as a public health problem.

In 2021, the WHO released a new guideline for on the pharmacological treatment of hypertension in adults. The publication provides evidence-based recommendations for the initiation of treatment of hypertension, and recommended intervals for follow-up. The document also includes target blood pressure to be achieved for control, and information on who, in the health-care system, can initiate treatment.

To support governments in strengthening the prevention and control of cardiovascular disease, WHO and the United States Centers for Disease Control and Prevention (U.S. CDC) launched the Global Hearts Initiative in September 2016, which includes the HEARTS technical package. The six modules of the HEARTS technical package (Healthy-lifestyle counselling,

Evidence-based treatment protocols, Access
to essential medicines and technology,
Risk-based management, Team-based care,
and Systems for monitoring) provide a
strategic approach to improve
cardiovascular health in countries across the
world.

In September 2017, WHO began a
partnership with Resolve to Save Lives, an
initiative of Vital Strategies, to support
national governments to implement the
Global Hearts Initiative. Other partners
contributing to the Global Hearts Initiative
are: the CDC Foundation, the Global Health
Advocacy Incubator, the Johns Hopkins
Bloomberg School of Public Health, the Pan
American Health Organization (PAHO) and
the U.S. CDC. Since implementation of the
programme in 2017 in 18 low- and
middle-income countries, 3 million people
have been put on protocol-based
hypertension treatment through
person-centred models of care. These

programmes demonstrate the feasibility and effectiveness of standardized hypertension control programmes.

Chapter 2: RISK FACTORS FOR HYPERTENSION

Modifiable and non-modifiable risk factors for hypertension

Hypertension, often referred to as high blood pressure (BP), is one of the most common yet silent chronic diseases that affects up to 1 in 3 adults in the United Kingdom. Despite being one of the biggest risk factors of cardiovascular disease, high BP is both preventable and manageable. We will explore some of the non-modifiable and modifiable risk factors of high BP.

Non-modifiable risk factors

Non-modifiable risk factors are factors that cannot be changed or adjusted, hence they are out of our control. These include:

Genetics

Having a family history of high BP means that someone within your immediate family has been diagnosed with high BP before the age of 60 years. The more family members that live with the condition, the greater the risk.

Age

As we age our risk of high BP increases. This is due to changes in the heart and blood vessels, whereby there is a loss of elasticity in the tissues found in our arteries. This loss of elasticity results in stiffening and a reduced ability to stretch, leading to increased BP.

Sex

More men are affected by high BP in early life, whereas after the age of 60 years more women have high BP. These differences are largely due to differing hormone profiles between men and women, and the hormonal changes associated with menopause.

Ethnicity

People of African and Black Caribbean descent have an increase in the risk of high BP . This is said to be down to genetic predisposition that increases sensitivity to salt in the diet by as little as 1 gram of extra salt per day can increase systolic BP, the pressure exerted on blood vessels when the heart contracts, by as little as much as 5mmHg; the unit of measurement that used when determining BP.

Modifiable risk factors

These are the factors that are in our control, including:

High salt diet

Excess dietary salt is one of the biggest risk factors for high BP. It is recommended adults in the UK consume no more than 6g per day, however the average intake is around 8g. Consuming too much salt causes the body to retain water to dilute the increased levels of salt which, in turn, increases BP.

Foods high in salt include:
Bread
Ready meals, such as pizza
Smoked and cured meats
Foods canned with added salt, such as beans
Adding table salt to meals and cooking

Body weight

Excess body weight increases the risk of high BP through several mechanisms. When an individual is overweight, the heart must work harder to pump blood around the body. Weight loss of 10kg can reduce systolic BP by as much as 5-20mmHg.

Smoking

Smoking just 1 cigarette can produce an immediate and temporary 5-10mmHg increase in BP. This is primarily due to the short- and long-term effects of nicotine in increasing heart rate and in the narrowing and hardening of arteries.

Exercise

Undertaking regular exercise helps to make our heart stronger, and a stronger heart can pump more blood more efficiently. It is recommended we undertake at least 150 minutes of moderate aerobic activity, such as walking, or 75 minutes of vigorous aerobic activity, such as jogging. Doing so can lower BP by as much as 5-8mmHg.

Stress

Stress is not necessarily a bad thing in and of itself. But too much stress may contribute to increased blood pressure. Also, too much stress can encourage behaviors that increase blood pressure, such as poor diet, physical inactivity, and using tobacco or drinking alcohol more than usual. Socioeconomic status and psychosocial stress can affect access to basic living necessities, medication, healthcare providers, and the ability to adopt healthy lifestyle changes.

When preexisting medical conditions cause high blood pressure

A small number of high blood pressure cases are **secondary hypertension** — high blood pressure that's caused by another medical condition that was present first. Examples include pregnancy-induced hypertension (PIH), certain heart defects, and kidney disorders. Most often, if the condition causing the high blood pressure can be resolved, the individual's blood pressure will normalize as well.

Chapter 3: COMPLICATIONS OF HYPERTENSION

Complications of hypertension are clinical complications that emerge from the chronic raising of blood pressure. Hypertension is a risk factor for all clinical symptoms of atherosclerosis since it is a risk factor for atherosclerosis itself. It is an independent predisposing factor for heart failure, coronary artery disease, stroke, kidney disease, and peripheral arterial disease. It is the most important risk factor for cardiovascular morbidity and mortality, in industrialized countries.

Complications affecting the heart

Left ventricular hypertrophy
Hypertensive heart disease is the outcome of structural and functional adaptations leading to left ventricular hypertrophy,

diastolic dysfunction, CHF, anomalies of blood flow due to atherosclerotic coronary artery disease and microvascular disease, and cardiac arrhythmias. Individuals with left ventricular hypertrophy are at increased risk for, stroke, CHF, and sudden death. Aggressive treatment of hypertension can regress or reverse left ventricular hypertrophy and lower the risk of cardiovascular disease. left ventricular hypertrophy is observed in 25% of hypertension patients and can easily be detected by utilizing echocardiography. Underlying processes of hypertensive left ventricular hypertrophy are of 2 types: mechanical, predominantly leading to myocyte enlargement; neuro-hormonal, mainly resulting in a fibroblastic proliferation.

Abnormalities of diastolic function, ranging from asymptomatic heart disease to overt heart failure, are common in hypertension patients. Patients with diastolic heart failure have a preserved ejection fraction, which is a marker of systolic function. Diastolic dysfunction is an early result of hypertension-related heart disease and is aggravated by left ventricular hypertrophy and ischemia.

Complications affecting the brain

Hypertensive Encephalopathy

Hypertension is a key risk factor for brain infarction and hemorrhage. Approximately 85% of strokes are due to infarction and the remainder is due to bleeding, either intracerebral hemorrhage or subarachnoid hemorrhage. The incidence of stroke grows progressively with increasing blood pressure levels, particularly systolic blood pressure in adults >65 years. Treatment of hypertension convincingly decreases the incidence of both ischemic and hemorrhagic strokes.

Hypertension is also connected with poorer cognition in the elderly population. Hypertension-related cognitive impairment and dementia may be a consequence of a single infarct due to occlusion of a "strategic" bigger vasculature or many lacunar infarcts due to occlusive small artery disease resulting in subcortical white matter ischemia. Several clinical trials suggest that antihypertensive medication has a favorable effect on cognitive function, however, this remains an active area of inquiry.

Cerebral blood flow remains unaltered over a wide range of arterial pressures (mean arterial pressure of 50–150 mmHg) by a process termed autoregulation of blood flow. Indications and symptoms of hypertensive encephalopathy may include severe headache, nausea and vomiting (sometimes of a projectile type), focal neurologic signs, and abnormalities in mental status. Untreated, hypertensive encephalopathy may develop into stupor, coma, seizures, and death within hours. It is important to distinguish hypertensive encephalopathy from other neurologic syndromes that may be associated with hypertension, e.g., cerebral ischemia, hemorrhagic or thrombotic stroke, seizure disorder, mass lesions, pseudotumor cerebri, delirium tremens, meningitis, acute intermittent porphyria, traumatic or chemical injury to the brain, and uremic encephalopathy.

Complications affecting the eye

Hypertensive retinopathy

Hypertensive retinopathy with AV nicking and moderate vascular tortuosity Hypertensive retinopathy is a disorder characterized by a spectrum of retinal vascular symptoms in persons with increased blood pressure. It was first described by Liebreich in 1859. The retinal circulation undergoes several pathophysiological alterations in response to high blood pressure. In the early, vasoconstrictive stage, there is vasospasm and a rise in retinal arteriolar tone attributable to local autoregulatory mechanisms. This stage is recognized clinically as a widespread constriction of the retinal arterioles. Persistently high blood pressure leads to intimal thickening, hyperplasia of the media wall, and hyaline degeneration in the subsequent, sclerotic, stage. This stage correlates to more severe generalized and focused areas of arteriolar narrowing, changes in the arteriolar and venular junctions, and variations in the arteriolar light reflex (i.e., widening and accentuation of the central light reflex, or "copper wire") (i.e., widening and accentuation of the central light reflex, or "copper wiring").

This is followed by an exudative stage, in which there is rupture of the blood-retina barrier, necrosis of the smooth muscles and endothelial cells, exudation of blood and lipids, and retinal ischemia. These alterations are exhibited in the retina as microaneurysms, hemorrhages, hard exudates, and cotton-wool patches. Swelling of the optic disk may develop at this time and usually signifies severely increased blood pressure (i.e., malignant hypertension) (i.e., malignant hypertension). Because better procedures for the regulation of blood pressure are now accessible in the general population, malignant hypertension is rarely found. In contrast, other retinal vascular consequences of hypertension, such as microaneurysms and branch-vein occlusions, are not uncommon in people with chronically increased blood pressure. These stages of hypertensive retinopathy, however, may not be sequential. For example, indications of retinopathy that represent the exudative stage, such as retinal hemorrhage or microaneurysm, may be found in eyes that do not contain hallmarks of the sclerotic stage, The exudative symptoms are general since they are seen in diabetes and other illnesses.

Complications affecting the kidneys

Hypertensive nephropathy

Hypertension is a risk factor for chronic kidney disease and end-stage kidney disease (ESKD) (ESKD). Kidney risk appears to be more closely associated with systolic than diastolic blood pressure, and black men are at greater risk than white men for developing ESRD at every level of blood pressure.

The atherosclerotic, hypertension-related vascular lesions in the kidney largely impact the preglomerular arterioles, resulting in ischemic alterations in the glomeruli and postglomerular structures. Glomerular injury may also be a consequence of direct damage to the glomerular capillaries due to glomerular hyperperfusion. The glomerular disease proceeds to glomerulosclerosis, and finally, the renal tubules may also become ischemic and gradually atrophic. The kidney lesion associated with malignant hypertension consists of fibrinoid necrosis of the afferent arterioles, sometimes extending into the glomerulus, and may result in focal necrosis of the glomerular tuft.

Clinically, macroalbuminuria (a random urine albumin/creatinine ratio > 300 mg/g) or microalbuminuria (a random urine albumin/creatinine ratio of 30–300 mg/g) are early indications of kidney impairment. These are also risk factors for kidney disease development and cardiovascular disease.

Complications connected to diabetes and hypertension

Diabetes has various problems of which one is hypertension or high blood pressure. Data reveal that at least 60-80 percent of those who get diabetes will later develop high blood pressure. High blood pressure is gradual in its early stages and may take at least 10–15 years to fully develop. Besides diabetes, additional variables that may contribute promote high blood pressure include obesity, insulin resistance, and high cholesterol levels. In general, fewer than 25 percent of diabetics have good control of their blood pressure. The prevalence of high blood pressure in diabetes is connected with a 4 fold risk of death mostly from heart disease and strokes. It has also been established in recent epidemiological research that fluctuation in blood pressure, independent of mean blood pressure level, contributes to microvascular and macrovascular problems in those with diabetes, including heart failure. These variable relationships may be especially detrimental in patients with either exceptionally high or particularly low blood pressures.

The major reason why patients with diabetes develop high blood pressure is the hardening of the arteries. Diabetes tends to speed up the progression of atherosclerosis. The other thing concerning diabetes is that it affects both major and tiny blood vessels in the body. Over time, blood arteries become clogged with fatty depots, become non-compliant, and lose their suppleness. The process of atherosclerosis is a lot faster in diabetic patients who do not have adequate control

of their blood glucose. High blood pressure eventually leads to heart failure, strokes, heart attacks, blindness, kidney failure, loss of libido, and poor circulation of blood in the legs. When the blood flow to the foot is weakened, the chances of infections and amputations also increase. All diabetics should recognize that even moderate rises in blood pressure can be hazardous to health. Studies have revealed that diabetics with even a minor rise in blood pressure have 2-3 times the risk of heart disease compared to persons without diabetes.

Blood pressure levels do fluctuate however specialists recommend that blood pressure should not range above 140/80. Secondly, high blood pressure is a silent condition and thus it is necessary for all diabetics to regularly check their blood pressure or have it checked at a doctor's office regularly. The American Diabetes Association recommends that all diabetics get their blood pressure tested by a health care practitioner at least 2-5 times a year.

Chapter 4: PREVENTION AND MANAGEMENT OF HYPERTENSION

An Overview of High Blood Pressure Treatment

Hypertension, or high blood pressure, is dangerous because it can lead to strokes, heart attacks, heart failure, or kidney disease. The goal of hypertension treatment is to lower high blood pressure and protect important organs, like the brain, heart, and kidneys from damage. Treatment for hypertension has been associated with reductions in stroke (reduced an average of 35%-40%), heart attack (20%-25%), and heart failure (more than 50%), according to research.

High blood pressure is now classified as a systolic blood pressure greater than 130 and diastolic over 80.

To prevent high blood pressure, everyone should be encouraged to make lifestyle modifications, such as eating a healthier diet, quitting smoking, and getting more exercise. Treatment with medication is recommended to lower blood pressure to less than 130/80 in people older than age 65 and those with risk factors such as diabetes and high cholesterol.

Treating high blood pressure involves lifestyle changes and possibly drug therapy.

•Lifestyle Changes to Treat High Blood Pressure

A critical step in preventing and treating high blood pressure is a healthy lifestyle. You can lower your blood pressure with the following lifestyle changes:

•**Losing weight** if you are overweight or obese

•**Quitting smoking.** Tobacco damages the walls of your blood vessels and hardens your arteries. Both need to be in good shape while you control your blood pressure.

•**Following the DASH eating plan, which stands for Dietary Approaches to Stop Hypertension.** It focuses on vegetables, fruits, whole grains fish, poultry, nuts, and beans. High-potassium foods, like avocados, bananas, dried fruits, tomatoes, and black beans, get a big thumbs-up. This plan keeps sugary drinks, sweets, and high-fat meats and dairy products at a minimum.

•**Reducing the amount of sodium in your diet to less than 1,500 milligrams a day** if you have high blood pressure; healthy adults should try to limit their sodium intake to no more than 2,300 milligrams a day (about 1 teaspoon of salt). Many processed foods have a lot of salt in them. For instance, soups, condiments, and tomato sauce can have as much as 75% of the total amount of salt you need each day. Read food labels carefully (salt is listed as sodium), and don't sprinkle more on when you cook or before you eat. Instead, use spices and herbs to flavor your food.

•**Getting regular aerobic exercise** (such as brisk walking at least 30 minutes a day, several days a week). Check out a yoga class. Seek out activities that get your heart pounding, like biking or swimming. Over the course of a week, aim to exercise consistently for at least 2 1/2 hours total.

•**Keeping a healthy weight for your age and height is key**. If you're overweight or have obesity, you can lower your blood pressure by losing just 5 pounds.

•**Limiting alcohol** to two drinks a day for men, one drink a day for women. One drink

is an ounce of alcohol, 5 ounces of wine, or
12 ounces of beer.

•**Reducing stress**. Think about stressful
areas of your life and take steps to change
them. Consider talking to a counselor,
learning meditation or anger-control
techniques, or getting regular massages.

In addition to lowering blood pressure,
many of these measures enhance the
effectiveness of high blood pressure drugs.

Drugs to Treat High Blood Pressure
There are several types of drugs used to
treat high blood pressure, including:

•Angiotensin-converting enzyme (ACE)
inhibitors
•Angiotensin II receptor blockers (ARBs)
•Diuretics
•Beta-blockers
•Calcium channel blockers

- Alpha-blockers
- Alpha-agonists
- Renin inhibitors
- Combination medications

Diuretics are often recommended as the first line of therapy for most people who have high blood pressure.

High Blood Pressure Treatment Follow-Up

The most important element in the management of high blood pressure is follow-up care.

- After starting high blood pressure drug therapy, you should see your doctor at least once a month until the blood pressure goal is reached. Once or twice a year, your doctor may check the level of potassium in your blood (diuretics can lower this, and ACE inhibitors and ARBs may increase this) and other electrolytes and BUN/creatinine levels (to check the health of the kidneys).

•After the blood pressure goal is reached, you should continue to see your doctor every 3 to 6 months, depending on whether you have other diseases such as heart failure.

•If you have diabetes or have had a heart attack or stroke, you'll need to keep a closer watch on your blood pressure to prevent recurrent events. Check with your doctor about what blood pressure readings you should be aiming for.

•With aging and hardening of the arteries, your systolic blood pressure may creep up. A treatment that once worked well may no longer work. Your drug dosage may need to be changed, or you may be prescribed a new medication.

•Periodically, at your follow-up visits, you should be screened for damage to the heart, eyes, brain, kidney, and peripheral arteries that may be related to high blood pressure.

•Follow-up visits are a good time to let your doctor know about any side effects you're having from your medication. They will have suggestions for coping with side effects or may change your treatment.

•Follow-up visits are a great opportunity for monitoring other associated risk factors, such as high cholesterol and obesity.

High Blood Pressure Drugs and How They Work

For most people, medication is a major part of the plan to lower their blood pressure. These drugs, also called "anti-hypertensive" medicine, won't cure high blood pressure. But they can help bring it back down to a normal range.

Which medicine you should take depends on things like:

i. How high your blood pressure is

ii. What's causing it

iii. How your body responds to the drugs

iv. Other health problems you have

Many people need more than one type of medication to control their high blood pressure. It may take some time working with your doctor to find the drugs and doses that work best for you.

Hypertensive drugs and their effect

Diuretics

These are often called **"water pills."** They're usually the first type of high blood pressure medicine that your doctor will try.

They help your kidneys take salt and water out of your body. Because you have less total fluid in your blood vessels, like a garden hose that's not turned on all the way, the pressure inside will be lower.

•Amiloride (Midamor)
•Bumetanide (Bumex)
•Chlorthalidone (Hygroton)
•Chlorothiazide (Diuril)
•Furosemide (Lasix)
•Hydrochlorothiazide or HCTZ (Esidrix, Hydrodiuril, Microzide)
•Indapamide (Lozol)
•Metolazone (Mykrox, Zaroxolyn)
•Spironolactone (Aldactone)
•Triamterene (Dyrenium)

Sometimes you can get more than one diuretic in a single pill.

•Amiloride + hydrochlorothiazide (Moduretic)

•Spironolactone + hydrochlorothiazide
(Aldactazide)
•Triamterene + hydrochlorothiazide
(Dyazide, Maxzide)

Beta-Blockers

They'll slow down your heartbeat and keep your heart from squeezing hard. This makes blood go through your vessels with less force.

•Acebutolol (Sectral)
•Atenolol (Tenormin)
•Betaxolol (Kerlone)
•Bisoprolol (Zebeta)
•Carteolol (Cartrol)
•Metoprolol (Lopressor, Toprol XL)
•Nadolol (Corgard)
•Nebivolol (Bystolic)
•Penbutolol (Levatol)
•Pindolol (Visken)
•Propranolol (Inderal)
•Sotalol (Betapace)

•Timolol (Blocadren)

Alpha-Blockers

These stop nerve signals before they can tell your blood vessels to tighten. Your vessels stay relaxed, giving the blood more room to move and lowering your overall blood pressure.

•Doxazosin (Cardura)
•Prazosin (Minipress)
•Terazosin (Hytrin)

ACE Inhibitors

Angiotensin-converting enzyme inhibitors prevent your body from making a hormone that tells blood vessels to tighten. With less of this hormone in your body, your blood vessels stay more open.

•Benazepril (Lotensin)
•Captopril (Capoten)
•Enalapril (Vasotec)

•Fosinopril (Monopril)
•Lisinopril (Prinivil, Zestril)
•Moexipril (Univasc)
•Perindopril (Aceon)
•Quinapril (Accupril)
•Ramipril (Altace)
•Trandolapril (Mavik)

ARBs

Angiotensin II receptor blockers stop that same hormone from working. Your body makes it, but ARBs prevent the hormone from constricting the muscles in your blood vessels, like putting chewing gum in a lock.

•Candesartan (Atacand)
•Eprosartan (Teveten)
•Irbesartan (Avapro)
•Losartan (Cozaar)
•Telmisartan (Micardis)
•Valsartan (Diovan)

Direct Renin Inhibitors

These target the same process that ACE inhibitors and ARBs do, so your blood vessels don't tighten up. But they work on the enzyme renin instead. They stop it from triggering reactions before the hormone gets made.

•Aliskiren (Tekturna) is a direct renin inhibitor.

Calcium Channel Blockers

They're sometimes called CCBs for short, or calcium antagonists. They don't let calcium into certain muscle cells in your heart and blood vessels, so it's harder for electrical signals to pass. Some CCBs keep blood vessels from tightening. Others slow your heart rate or make your heart ease up on how hard it squeezes to push blood.

•Amlodipine (Norvasc)
•Bepridil (Vasocor)

•Diltiazem (Cardizem, Dilacor, Tiazac)
•Felodipine (Plendil)
•Isradipine (DynaCirc)
•Nicardipine (Cardene)
•Nifedipine (Adalat, Procardia)
•Nisoldipine (Sular)
•Verapamil (Calan, Covera, Isoptin, Verelan)

Central Agonists

They stop your brain from sending signals that speed up your heart rate and narrow your blood vessels. These drugs are also called central-acting agents, central adrenergic inhibitors, and central alpha agonists.

•Clonidine (Catapres)
•Guanabenz (Wytensin)
•Guanfacine (Tenex)
•Methyldopa (Aldomet)

Peripheral Adrenergic Blockers

They prevent signals that your brain sends from getting to your blood vessels and telling them to tighten. Doctors don't prescribe these drugs often.

- Guanadrel (Hylorel)
- Guanethidine (Ismelin)
- Reserpine (Serpasil)

Vasodilators

These relax the muscles in your blood vessel walls. The vessels widen, and blood can flow through more easily.

- Hydralazine (Apresoline)
- Minoxidil (Loniten)

Combinations

Some medicines combine different kinds of drugs.

•Bisoprolol + hydrocholorthiazide (Ziac), beta-blocker and diuretic
•Carvedilol (Coreg), alpha-blocker and beta-blocker
•Labetalol (Normodyne, Trandate), alpha-blocker and beta-blocker
•Olmesartan + hydrocholorthiazide (Benicar), ARB and diuretic

Chapter 5: DASH DIET AND HYPERTENSION

One of the steps your doctor may recommend to lower your high blood pressure is to start using the DASH diet.

DASH stands for Dietary Approaches to Stop Hypertension (high blood pressure). The diet is simple:

•Eat more fruits, vegetables, and low-fat dairy foods

•Cut back on foods that are high in saturated fat, cholesterol, and trans fats

•Eat more whole-grain foods, fish, poultry, and nuts

•Limit sodium, sweets, sugary drinks, and red meats

In research studies, people who were on the DASH diet lowered their blood pressure within 2 weeks.

Another diet -- DASH-Sodium -- calls for cutting back sodium to 1,500 milligrams a day (about 2/3 teaspoon). Studies of people on the DASH-Sodium plan lowered their blood pressure as well.

Starting the DASH Diet

The DASH diet calls for a certain number of servings daily from various food groups. The number of servings you require may vary, depending on how many calories you need per day.

You can make gradual changes. For instance, start by limiting yourself to 2,400 milligrams of sodium per day (about 1 teaspoon). Then, once your body has adjusted to the diet, cut back to 1,500 milligrams of sodium per day (about 2/3 teaspoon). These amounts include all sodium eaten, including sodium in food products as well as in what you cook with or add at the table.

Dash Diet Tips

•Add a serving of vegetables at lunch and at dinner.

•Add a serving of fruit to your meals or as a snack. Canned and dried fruits are easy to use, but check that they don't have added sugar.

•Use only half your typical serving of butter, margarine, or salad dressing, and use low-fat or fat-free condiments.

•Drink low-fat or skim dairy products any time you would normally use full-fat or cream.

•Limit meat to 6 ounces a day. Make some meals vegetarian.

•Add more vegetables and dry beans to your diet.

•Instead of snacking on chips or sweets, eat unsalted pretzels or nuts, raisins, low-fat and fat-free yogurt, frozen yogurt, unsalted plain popcorn with no butter, and raw vegetables.

•Read food labels to choose products that are lower in sodium.

Staying on the DASH Diet
The DASH diet suggests getting:

Grains: 7-8 daily servings

Vegetables: 4-5 daily servings

Fruits: 4-5 daily servings

Low-fat or fat-free dairy products: 2-3 daily servings

Meat, poultry, and fish: 2 or less daily servings

Nuts, seeds, and dry beans: 4-5 servings per week

Fats and oils: 2-3 daily servings

Sweets: try to limit to less than 5 servings per week

How Much Is a Serving?

When you're trying to follow a healthy eating plan, it helps to know how much of a certain kind of food is considered a "serving." One serving is:

- •1/2 cup cooked rice or pasta
- •1 slice bread

•1 cup raw vegetables or fruit
•1/2 cup cooked veggies or fruit
•8 ounces of milk
•1 teaspoon of olive oil (or any other oil)
•3 ounces cooked meat
•3 ounces tofu